Meat Stock and Bone Broth:

The Health and Healing Effect of Meat Stock and Bone Broth

Table of Contents

Introduction

Thanks and congratulations for downloading *Meat Stock and Bone Broth: The Health and Healing Effect of Meat Stock and Bone Broth.* When it comes to a single change that can lead to the greatest number of long term positive results, bone broth and meat stock are without a doubt at the top of the list. Long considered super foods, these two similar nutritional delicacies are good for what ails you when it comes to digestive issues, guaranteed. If you are having issues already, it is best to start with meat stock, otherwise jumping straight to bone broth is acceptable.

This book contains proven steps and strategies designed to ensure you learn everything you need to about just what goodness bone broth and meat stock are putting into your body. You will also find tips for finding the best bones, ways to ensure your bone broth and meat stock is as healthy as possible, and recipes that can be used for practically every type of meat and bone available.

Thanks again for choosing this book, let's hope you like what you read!

Chapter 1: Bone Broth Benefits

Despite having fallen out of favor in the United States over the past few generations, bone broth is still consumed worldwide in much the same way as it has been for thousands and thousands of years. This is in part due to the ready availability of the primary ingredients, partially in part to the ease with which the ingredients can be modified based on availability and almost certainly largely because of the high nutrient content the brew contains. So many nutrients, in fact, that it can be said that homemade bone broth is one of the most nutritious things you can put in your body.

Humanity has been wise to the vital nutrients that are hidden in the bones of the animals they eat since the species as a whole had yet to discover agriculture. The scarcity inherent in the lifestyle meant that nothing, not even the knuckle or hoof bones were thrown away, and instead, they were burned. When the bones were thrown into the fire, something amazing happened, the heat brought out the nutrients that were hidden in these bones and their delicious taste emphasized their healthy nature.

The process of heating bones to maximize their nutrients continued, and as the process became refined over time, boiling the bones became the process du jour when it came to getting the most out of each leftover bone's nutrients.

Perhaps unsurprisingly, the parts of the world which still include a hearty helping of bone broth in their diet, as well as things like vegetables, complex carbohydrates and healthy fats are known to have a much lower risk of cancer, heart disease and stroke, especially when compared with the diet of the average American.

All told, bone broth has been recommended for regular consumption by notable figures throughout history such as the great Grecian doctor Hippocrates, Maimonides, the ancient philosopher and even Charlemagne himself. South America proverb states it best perhaps when it notes that when the quality is high enough, bone broth is so healthy it can wake the dead.

Just what makes it so nutritious?

Bone Marrow: While bone marrow is traditionally thought of as a single thing, in reality it is split between what is known as red marrow and what is known as yellow marrow. All marrow begins as red marrow and then yellows over time until roughly 50 percent of the total is yellow. Red marrow is known to contain high amounts of vitamins and nutrients while yellow marrow is known to be a great source of healthy fats and lipids. Red marrow is commonly found in flat bones and hip bones as well as in the sternum, scapula, skull, ribs and vertebrae. These bones also contain elements that are crucial for making sure oxygen moves through the body as it should while also making open cuts clot faster.

Cartilage: This is most commonly found in joints and is known to break down when cooked into broth and, in turn, improve the strength of the individual cells it reacts with. In addition, it can lead to lower cholesterol which means lower risk of heart attack as well. It also improves the ability of blood vessels to maximize oxygen flow and minimize the swelling and pain typically associated with arthritis of many types.

Collagen: Once it has been removed from the bones via the cooking process, collagen becomes gelatin. Approximately one fourth of all of the protein in the body is tied up in collagen, bone marrow, cartilage, bones, tendons and skin. Consuming regular amount of gelatin is important to ensure your intestines are well coated which helps prevent cuts or tears from forming while also reducing inflammation throughout the body.

Minerals: While numerous minerals are released into the broth during the cooking process, there are three big ones that are crucial to receive in regular doses for maximum health benefits. First of all, calcium is important to ensuring ideal muscle function, helping cuts heal quickly and keeping bones nice and hearty. Phosphorus is crucial to ensuring your body produces the amount of energy it needs to work properly and magnesium is critical for keeping your enzymes and nerves working properly.

Additional health benefits
With so much nutrition practically bursting from the seams, is it any wonder that the benefits of consuming bone broth regularly reach literally from head to toe? Consider the following reasons to give it a try:

- *Improve intestinal health:* Studies show that as little as 8 oz. of bone broth per day is enough to improve overall digestive tract health and can even go so far as to complete stop leaky gut syndrome symptoms from appearing. This is thanks to the gelatin in the broth which can actually patch holes in the gut as it moves through it. As a side effect of this process, instances of diarrhea, constipation and food intolerance should all naturally decrease as well.

- *Improve joints:* The glucosamine found in bone broth goes a long way towards naturally mitigating pain that can commonly occur in the joints while at the same time improving their health as well, especially when paired with all that gelatin. Chondroitin sulfate, also is known to appear in bone broth in large quantities, is a direct inhibitor to the expressed symptoms of osteoarthritis.

- *Create healthier skin:* Collagen is an important component to keeping skin looking as tight and healthy as possible. As little as 8 ounces of bone broth consumed regularly can provide your skin with all the collagen it needs to looks its best in any situation. With enough additional collagen, you may even see an actually decrease in existing wrinkles in addition to simply preventing new ones from forming.

- *Improve your sleep cycle:* The glycine found in many types of bones can help regulate and moderate sleep cycles and improve the restorative effects of sleep when consumed regularly, such as by consuming a cup of bone broth per day for example. Glycine is also known to increase the memory and enhance focus.

- *It's a literal superfood:* A superfood is any naturally occurring food which contains a wide range of nutrients in amounts much higher than the average. This describes bone broth to the letter, it is the reason that chicken soup has always been known to cure the common cold. Ounce for once it is healthier than milk, even providing more of magnesium and phosphorus that ensure your bones stay healthy and strong.

- *It provides a real energy boost:* While scientists can't quite explain why it happens, anecdotally nearly everyone who tries it reports an almost immediate burst of energy akin to drinking a shot of espresso. The most likely explanation is that it is simply a positive side effect from consuming so many nutrients at once.

Full of healthy nutrients

Outside of all of these immediately noticeable benefits, bones are known to be a terrific source for protein comprising as much as roughly 50 percent of the bones total weight. This is a combination of the protein found in collagen as well as gelatin and a group of amino acids containing glycine and proline. Together, proline and glycine allow the body to repair the types of tissue that cause muscles to attach to bone and help to stop injuries from occurring. What this means is that if you are looking for a snack before the gym, you could do a whole lot worse than bone broth as it will help you train longer and harder without fear of injury.

In addition, studies show that common proteins found in bone broth are likely to provide significant relief to people suffering from rheumatoid arthritis. These proteins serve to mitigate the response from the autoimmune system which triggers the spread of the disease. Bone broth is so effective at mitigating the symptoms associated with the disease, in fact, that a recent study of more than 100 individuals with the disease saw a 100 percent reduction in the symptoms presented as well as a 75 percent success rate when it comes to sending the disease into total remission. What's more, these exact proteins are also known to work on other long lasting disease that are known to effect the autoimmune system as well.

Bone broth is useful when it comes to promoting joint health because of the obvious, but also because it contains several important types of glycosaminoglycan which are known to help improve the strength of connective tissue which means it is great for reducing inflammation and pain in unwieldy joints. Another type of glycosaminoglycan is hyaluronic acid; it is known to protect against the onset of osteoarthritis in joints throughout the body despite only being taken orally.

In addition, chondroitin sulfate, another type of glycosaminoglycan, is effective when it comes to repairing and reducing the long term damage often associated with arthritis. This glycosaminoglycan works with perhaps the most well-known variety, glucosamine which is commonly found in all types of joint health supplements. Glucosamine decreases pain and reduce joint inflammation symptoms. If you have ever had any type of joint issues, then a cup of bone broth each day will likely be quite good for what ails you.

Besides improving joint function and health, drinking bone broth on the regular is going to help your digestive tract significantly as well. Glycine is also useful in this instance as it will guarantee a more sustain and normal stomach acid flow which is sure to help digestion as well. Glycine pops up again as the primary ingredient in bile which is crucial to decreasing the overall level of fat in the intestines while also lowering negative cholesterol levels.

The restorative benefits found in bone broth are also known to combine in such a way that those who consume it regularly while recovering from a major injury have been known to recover almost 20 percent faster than those with the same injury who did not consume bone broth. This is thanks in part to the high amount of amino acids found in bone broth, amino acids that the body needs during serious bouts of self-repair in extremely high amounts.

Two additional nutrients that also help to maximizing the healing process are known as glutamine and arginine. Both nutrients are great at supporting bone health as well as tissue growth by increasing the amount of collagen the body produces which means that they also help reduce the visibility of scars.

Bone broth's restorative benefits have also been proven to extend to improving the ability to relax while also mitigating small pains or aches because glycine, once again, is also what is known as a neurotransmitter inhibitor. It also removes toxins that may be harmful to the liver from the body and also tackles fat that might be stored there. Finally, it also increases the amount of glutathione acid in the body which improvise antioxidant production.

Increases levels of glutathione are known to be directly related to the amount of vitamin C found in the body which also improves oxidation. It is also known to balance out the amount of methionine found in the body which is an important component when it comes to maintaining steady blood and vitamin B levels.

Don't forget about the marrow
The numerous health benefits discussed above have all been exclusively discussed with just the nutrients in the bone themselves being taken into account. Bone marrow is useful when it comes to helping to strengthen the immune system while also introducing numerous helpful types of cells into the body which are known to enhance immune response and improve the strength of bones. Marrow is also full of a distinct grouping of minerals depending on what type of animal they were once a part of. Fish bones are known to typically contain high quantities of iodine, fowl bones are known to be high in potassium and calcium, pork bones are rich in potassium and magnesium as are cow bones.

While every batch of broth is different because no two bones are exactly the same, a reliable rule as to the nutrition found within states that the better the animal was treated when it was alive, the more nutritious its bones will ultimately be. Aside from that, if you are looking to ensure each batch of broth is as nutritious as possible, it is important to make sure to include at least 1 tablespoon of something acidic to help the bones dissolve as fully as possible into the broth.

Additionally, you may want to consume the small bones which will be chewy and easy to eat after they have been cooked, some will even dissolve on your tongue. If you aren't interested in eating the bones directly, you can instead grind them up and then add the powder back into the broth directly. This should be done before the broth has had time to cool for the best results.

Chapter 2: Bone Broth Recipes

When it comes to making your own bone broth, finding the right bones for the job is often considered the hardest part. If you aren't sure where to find the types of bones you are looking for, one of the best places to start is the butcher section of a local grocery chain or possibly an Asian market. When it comes to choosing bones, it is important to remember that the tougher a bone is, the more full of nutrients it is likely to be. This means that you want to look for soup bones, chicken necks, beef knuckles, oxtails and chicken's feet.

Remember, aim for grass-fed animals whenever possible as they are going to be the healthiest options as a rule. If you are looking to find only bones that have been grass-fed exclusively then companies such as US Wellness Meats and Tropical Traditions are good places to start.

When it comes to storing your broth, it is important to start by cooling it as soon as it has finished cooking and then immediately place it is an airtight container in the freezer for the best results. You will want to do this with any broth you are not planning to eat for more than 3 days to keep it tasting its best for as long as possible. Always heat cold broth thoroughly and stir well to ensure each cup is as full of nutrients as possible.

Bone Broth Template

No matter the bones, this template can be used to make nutritious and delicious broth

What to Use
- Bones (2 lbs. your choice)
- Something acidic (apple cider vinegar 1 T)
- Vegetables (to taste)

What to Do
- Start by roasting the bones with the vegetables to maximize the flavor of each. Common vegetable choices include garlic, onions, pepper, salt and appropriate herbs.
- Add everything to a slow cooker before filling it with cold water
- Mix in the vinegar for the most nutritious results.
- Set the slow cooker on a low heat and let it cook for anywhere between 1 and 2 days for the best results. Chicken bones should be simmered for a minimum of 4 hours, beef bones should be cooked at least 6 and pork bones should be cooked a minimum of 8. Fish bones can be cooked for a minimum of 4 hours and a maximum of 24 hours.

Bone Broth-Chicken

One cup of this broth will be enough to convince you of store bought chicken soup's inferiority. This recipe results in approximately 8 cups of broth.

What to Use
- Chicken Bones (4 lbs.)
- Apple cider vinegar (1 T)
- Thyme (to taste)
- Parsley (to taste)
- Carrots (3 chopped)
- Celery (3 stalks chopped)
- Peppercorn (2 T)
- Garlic (1 clove minced)
- Onions (2)
- Bay leaf (1)

What to Do
- A slow cooker that is at least 6 quarts will provide you with enough room for the ingredients as well as the required water of 2.5 quarts.
- Make sure your oven is heated and ready at 400 degrees Fahrenheit
- Place the chicken bones on a baking sheet along with the thyme, parsley, carrots, celery, peppercorn, garlic, onions and bay leaf.
- Place the baking sheet in the oven and allow it to cook for 20 minutes before turning the pan 180 degrees and letting it bake for another 15 minutes.
- Remove the sheet from the oven before adding its contents to the slow cooker and seasoning as desired.
- Add in the apple cider vinegar and mix well before covering the slow cooker, and turning it on high long enough for the water to boil before turning the heat

to low and letting it cook for up to 4 hours.

Bone Broth-Beef
This broth definitely benefits from roasting the vegetables beforehand, give it a try and you won't ever want to go back. This recipe results in approximately 8 cups of broth.

What to Use
- Beef Bones (4 lbs.)
- Apple cider vinegar (1 T)
- Carrots (2)
- Bay leaf (2)
- Leek (1)
- Onion (1)
- Garlic (1 clove minced)
- Celery (2 stalks chopped)
- Black pepper (2 T)

What to Do
- A slow cooker that is at least 6 quarts will provide you with enough room for the ingredients as well as the required water of 2.5 quarts.
- Make sure your oven is heated and ready at 450 degrees Fahrenheit
- Place the beef bones on a baking sheet along with the garlic, carrots, onion and leek.
- Place the baking sheet in the oven and allow it to cook for 20 minutes before tossing the pan and letting it bake for another 15 minutes.

- Remove the sheet from the oven before adding its contents to the slow cooker and seasoning as desired.
- Add in the apple cider vinegar and mix well before covering the slow cooker, and turning it on high long enough for the water to boil before turning the heat to low and letting it cook for up to 4 hours.

Bone Broth-Pork

When it comes to making bone broth on the cheap, pork bones are often about half the price of beef bones. It is important to always strain this broth multiple times before freezing and again each time after it has been heated. This recipes yields approximately 2 quarts broth.

What to use
- Pork bones (3 lbs.)
- Apple cider vinegar (1 T)
- Ground black pepper (to taste)
- Sea salt (to taste)

What to do
- A slow cooker that is at least 6 quarts will provide you with enough room for the ingredients as well as the required water of 2.5 quarts.
- Add in all of the ingredients and let the slow cooker boil before setting the temperature to low and letting it cook for up to 48 hours.

Bone Broth- Fish

White fish is typically preferred when it comes to broth. Always include the heads as well as the fins in any fish broth, eyes are optional. This recipe will create approximately 8 cups of broth.

What to use
- Fish bones (2 lbs.)
- Apple cider vinegar (.25 cups)
- Sea salt (as needed)

What to do
- This recipe requires a slow cooker that is at least 4 quarts.
- Add in all of the ingredients as well as 3 quarts of water.
- Let the slow cooker boil and wait until a foam rises to the top of the water. Remove this foam as it is made of impurities in the fish that are leaving during the boiling process.
- Once the foam has been removed, cover the slow cooker, turn the heat to low and let it cook for no more than 24 hours.

Chapter 3: Meat Stock Benefits

While many people use the term meat stock and bone broth interchangeably, the two actually have a number of distinctions, especially when it comes to using them to improve any issue you might have with your digestive tract. Oddly enough, in the culinary world, stock is made from bones and broth is made from meat, nevertheless, the opposite is true when it comes to healthy eating. Primarily, meat stock is higher in the amino acids glycine and proline as well as gelatin which make it more beneficial when you are looking to actively heal digestive issues including leaky gut as the more gelatin you can get into your system in that situation the better. From there, bone broth is better when you are looking to maintain a healthy system. Additionally, meat stock is not cooked for as long as bone broth is.

Unique benefits
While cooking, the gelatinous protein found in the connective tissues of the meat that is being cooked are pulled into the stock, making it great for strengthening and healing the connective tissue of those who consume it. In addition, properly prepared stock promotes the proper moderation of hydrochloric acid in the system which also improves the overall digestive process by improving the rate at which proteins are broken down in the stomach. In fact, having too little hydrochloric

acid in stomach is known to cause food allergies as well as asthma, vitiligo, rheumatoid arthritis, osteoporosis, anemia, skin disorders, acid reflux disease and more.

The large amounts gelatin found in meat stock, even when taken in comparison to bone broth, makes it ideal for children and young adults to eat daily as it helps to ensure they continue to grow properly by receiving the vitamins and nutrients they need most. The higher level of gelatin is also good for making it easier for the human body to break down legumes as well as a myriad of grains that many people naturally have a difficult time processing properly. Meat stock is also suggested in place of bone broth in those who have ADHD, autism, or suffer from ticks or seizures as these individuals need to avoid glutamine, found in higher amounts in bone broth, which is known to exacerbate their symptoms.

Additional indications that you might want to stick with meat stock as opposed to bone broth is if you are exhibiting symptoms related to nervous system agitation or if your digestive tract is exhibiting issues expressing themselves as rashes, skin eruptions, constipation, nausea, vomiting or diarrhea.

Introduction to GAPS
Meat stock is also a key component of a diet designed to treat what is known as Gut and Psychology Syndrome a disease that manifests itself via numerous inflammatory and bowel related issues as well as other gastrointestinal

issues and systemic diseases. The goal of the diet is to reduce serious issues of gastrointestinal distress and initiate the natural healing process, primarily through the introduction of meat stock into the diet.

The idea here is that stock made from fish or meat will provide the cells of the lining of the digestive tract the building blocks they need to come back stronger and better than ever before. They also spread out and lead to a general soothing of the areas that see the most inflammation in target areas.

When it comes to getting the most out of meat stock, it is important to always make your own and never used store bought options as they are likely going to be extremely lacking when it comes to meaningful nutrients. Those following the GAPS diet find that chicken stock is the type of stock that is good for soothing even the most violently ill digestive tracts.

Chapter 4: Meat Stock Recipes

Making your own meat stock is quite similar to making bone broth, though there are a few differences. The biggest one of these is the drastically reduced cooking time when it comes to stock recipes as it is all about cooking the meat thoroughly without over cooking it. This means chicken will be cooked for 90 minutes, beef will be cooked for roughly 180 minutes and fish will be cooked for 60 minutes. Despite the shorter cooking times, however, the results from the stock recipes are likely to gel much more easily as they are full of quite a bit more fat as well.

To make the best stock you will want to seek out joint bones that still contain plenty of meat. Whole pheasants, ducks, turkeys or chickens will also work, though it is important to retain a focus on joints and bones. Try and include tubular bones that have been cut in half for easier access to the bone marrow for an extra healthy treat. Remember, in these situations, the quality of the cut of the meat doesn't matter nearly as much as the quality of the animal as a whole.

When it comes to utilizing the finished stock effectively, there is literally no wrong answer for this versatile food stuff. You can remove the meat from the bones and make a soup, and bone broth for good measure, or you can use it as the base for a vegetable broth or even drink it plain for a delicious pick me up at any time of the day. It can even be used as a based to glaze legumes or grains that your system otherwise has a hard time tolerating. The only thing that matter is that you are drinking it regularly and that you stick with it long enough for the practice to become habit.

Meat Stock Template
This stock is the basis of the introductory GAPS diet and will hit the spot if you are suffering from numerous types of intestinal trouble. It requires 5 minutes to prepare, 3 hours to cook and makes 16 cups.

What to Use
- Meat on the bone (2 lbs.)
- Water (16 cups filtered)

What to Do
- Add the meat and bones to a large stock pot before adding in the water, ensuring that it is enough to completely cover the bones.
- Place the stockpot on the stove over a burner set to a high/medium heat and let the meat cook for 3 hours.
- Run the results through a strainer to capture the broth directly. Save the rest of the ingredients for later consumption.
- Store in an airtight, glass container in the refrigerator for up to 4 days or in the freezer for 2 months.

Fish Meat Stock
This recipe can be made with any common fish that is not overly oily, sole is a good

substitution for the snapper. It requires 5 minutes to prepare, 1 hour to cook and makes 16 cups.

What to Use
- Snapper (2)
- Water (16 cups filtered)
- Raw apple cider vinegar (2 T)
- Celery (3 stalks chopped)
- Carrots (3 chopped)
- Yellow onions (2 medium chopped)
- Bay leaf (1)
- Sage (as needed dried, crushed)
- Rosemary (as needed dried, crushed)
- Thyme (as needed dried, crushed)
- Celtic Sea Salt (1.5 tsp.)
- Parsley (dried, crushed)

What to Do
- Using purified water, rinse the fish before remove the meat from the bones and reserve for use later.
- In a large stockpot, add in the heads, skin, tails, fins and bones as well as any thyme, rosemary, sage, bay, onions, celery, carrots and raw apple cider vinegar.
- Fill the stockpot with the 4 quarts of water before letting all of the ingredients sit for 90 minutes.
- Add the stockpot to the stove over a burner set to a high heat and let it boil before reducing the heat and letting it simmer for 90 minutes.

- 10 minutes before the stock has finished cooking, add in the salt as well as the parsley.
- Strain the stock prior to cooling or serving, fattier stocks will need a sturdy wire strainer.

Chicken Meat Stock

This recipe is also good for turkey, pheasant or any other type of fowl. This is widely considered the best stock when it comes to being mild on inflamed digestive tracts. It requires 5 minutes to prepare, 90 minutes to cook and makes 16 cups.

What to Use
- Chicken (1 whole)
- Chicken feet (2 optional)
- Chicken head (1 optional)
- Purified water (4 quarts)
- Apple cider vinegar (2 T)
- Yellow onions (2 chopped)
- Carrots (4 chopped)
- Celery (3 stalks chopped)
- Bouquet garni (1 tied with cooking twine)
- Bay leaf (1)
- Sage (2 tsp. dried, crushed)
- Rosemary (2 tsp. dried, crushed)
- Thyme (2 tsp. dried, crushed)
- Salt (2 tsp.)
- Parsley (2 tsp. dried, crushed)

What to Do

- Start by rinsing the various parts of the chicken in water that has been purified before cutting the chicken in half lengthwise.
- Place the various chicken pieces into a stockpot before adding in the thyme, rosemary, sage, bay, bouquet garni, carrots, yellow onions and vinegar. Season as desired.
- Add in the water and let everything sit for 30 minutes to give the apple cider vinegar time to do its thing.
- Add the pot to the stove over a burner turned to a high heat before letting it boil. Reduce the heat and allow the pot to simmer for 90 minutes.
- 10 minutes before the stock has finished cooking, add in the salt as well as the parsley.
- Strain the stock prior to cooling or serving and save the results for another meal. Remember, fattier stocks will need a sturdy wire strainer.

Beef Meat Stock
This recipe is just as delicious if you substitute lamb for beef. It is important to avoid adding starches to your stocks if you are looking to help mitigate digestive tract issues. It requires 5 minutes to prepare, 180 minutes to cook and makes 16 cups.

What to Use
- Purified water (4 quarts)
- Apple cider vinegar (2 T)
- Salt (2 tsp.)

- Parsley (2 tsp. dried, crushed)
- Garlic (1 clove crushed)
- Ginger (1 tsp.)
- Lemon rind (2 tsp. ground)
- Yellow onions (2 chopped)
- Carrots (4 chopped)
- Celery (3 stalks chopped)
- Bouquet garni (1 tied with cooking twine)
- Meaty ribs (3 lbs.)
- Bone marrow (2 lbs.)
- Knuckle bones (2 lbs.)

What to Do
- Roast the bones prior to making a stock for the best results.
- Add the knuckle bones, bone marrow, meaty ribs, bouquet garni, celery, carrots, yellow onions, lemon rind, ginger, apple cider vinegar and garlic to a large stockpot.
- Add in the water and let everything sit for 30 minutes to give the apple cider vinegar time to do its thing.
- Add the pot to the stove over a burner turned to a high heat before letting it boil. Reduce the heat and allow the pot to simmer for 180 minutes.
- 10 minutes before the stock has finished cooking, add in the salt as well as the parsley.
- Strain the stock prior to cooling or serving and save the results for another meal. Remember, fattier stocks will need a sturdy wire strainer.

Conclusion

Thank you again for downloading this book! I hope this book was able to help you to learn everything you wanted to know when it comes to the myriad of benefits that are available by simply drinking bone broth or meat stock regularly. Remember, the recipes in the preceding chapters are just a framework, add in your favorite bones and mix things up in the way that's right for you.

The next step is to stop reading already, break out the slow cooker and start making meat stock, if you have digestive issues, or bone broth if you are interested in making sure you continue not to have them. Make a conscious effort to drink it every day for a month and you will be shocked and pleased by the results. So much so that you won't ever want to go back.

Finally, if you enjoyed this book, or found it helpful in any way, then a review saying as much on Amazon would be extremely appreciated.